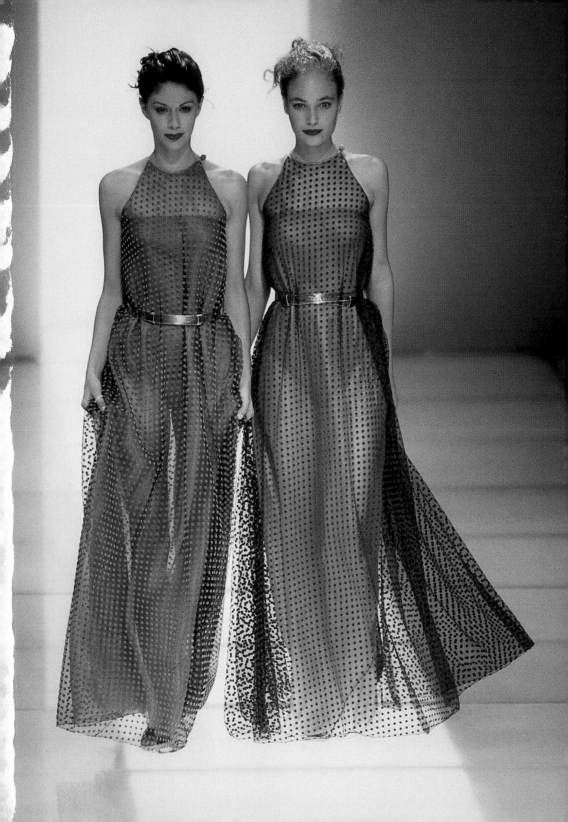

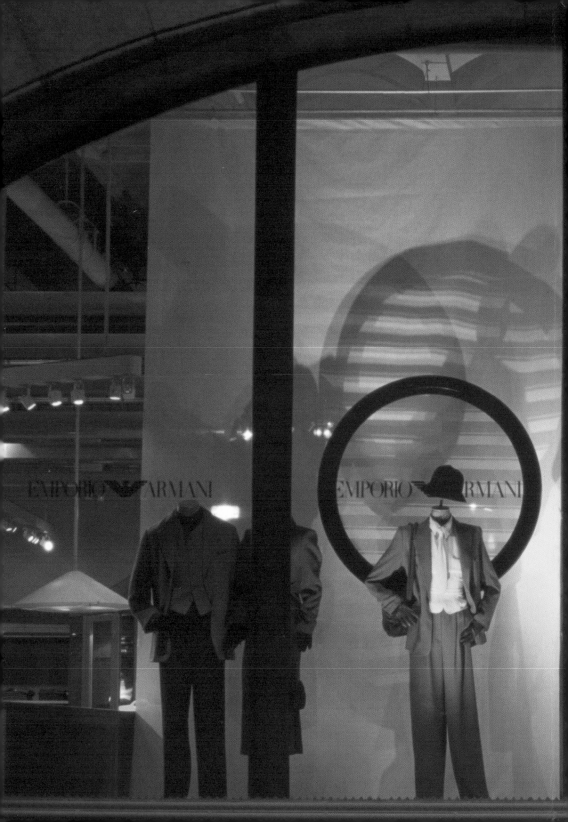

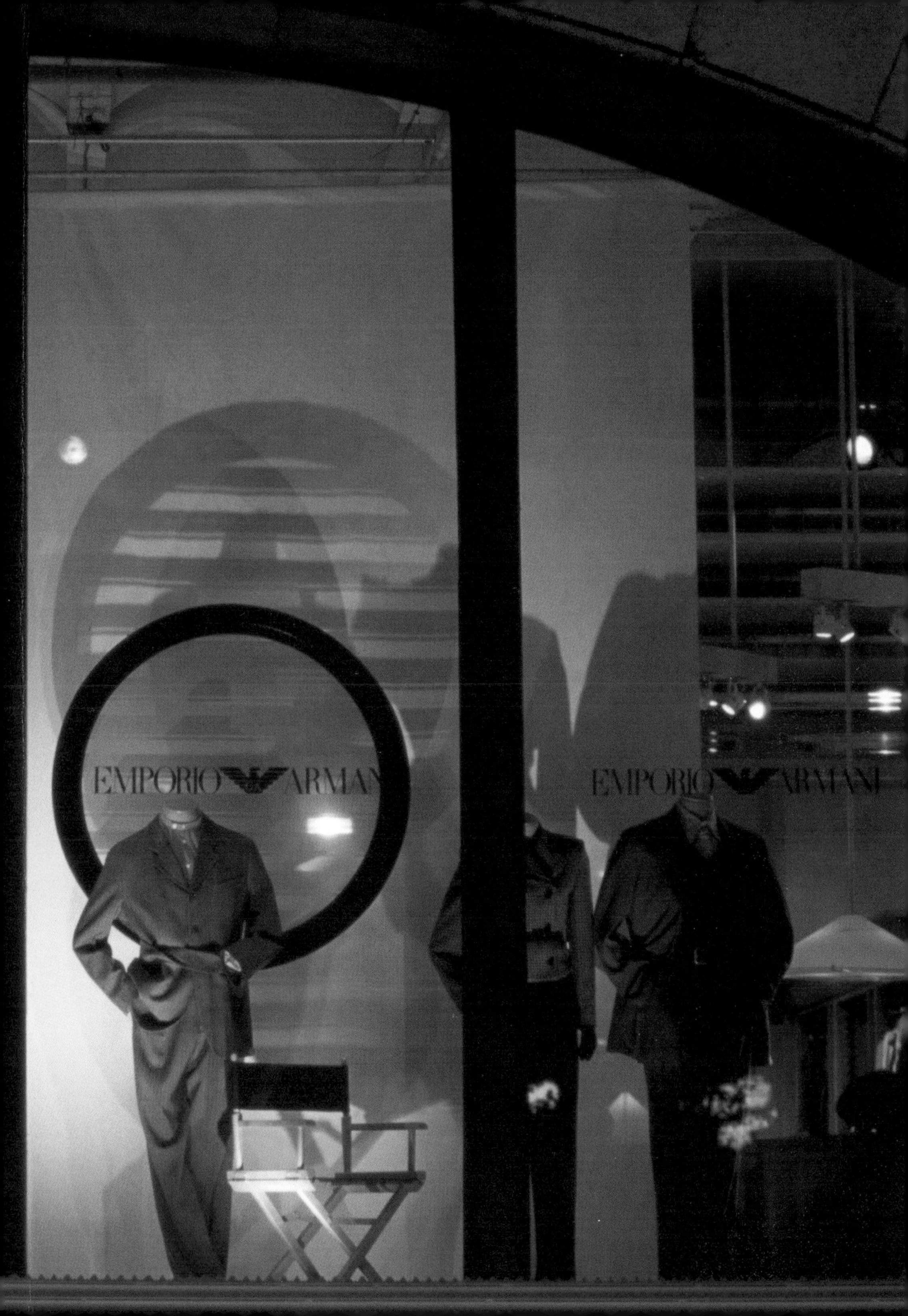
EMPORIO ARMANI
EMPORIO ARMANI

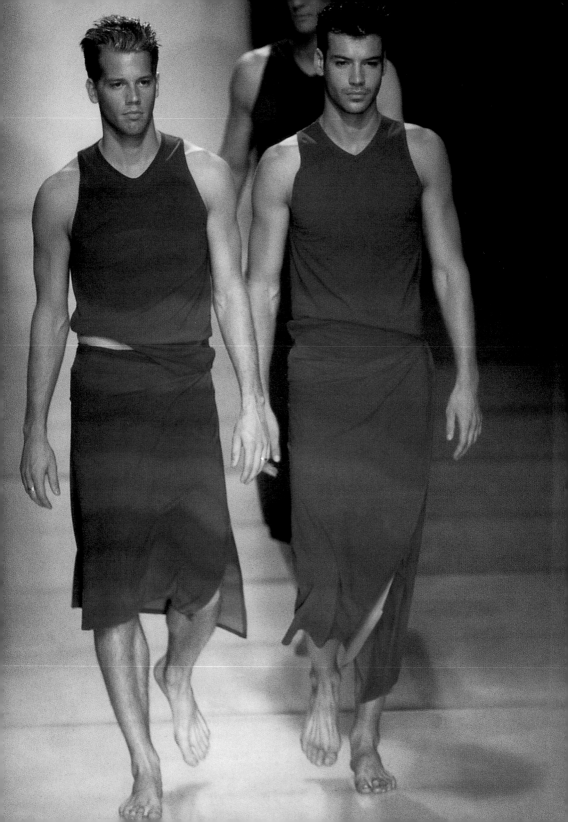

GIORGIO
Armani

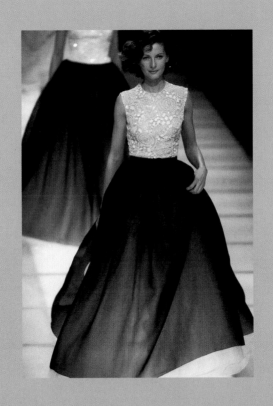

FOR CHRISTOPHER

THIS IS A CARLTON BOOK

Text and design copyright © 2000 Carlton Books Limited

This edition published by Carlton Books Limited 2000
20 Mortimer Street
London
W1N 7RD

A CIP catalogue for this book is available from the Library-of-Congress.

ISBN 1 85868 990 2

Project Editor: Camilla MacWhannell
Art Editor: Adam Wright
Design: Zoë Mercer
Picture research: Abi Dillon
Production: Janette Davis

Printed and bound in Dubai

GIORGIO
Armani

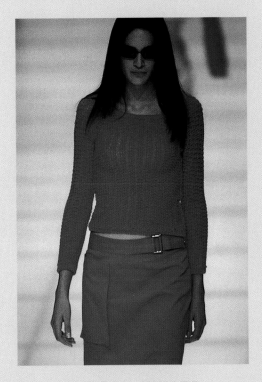

NICOLA WHITE

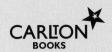

CARLTON
BOOKS

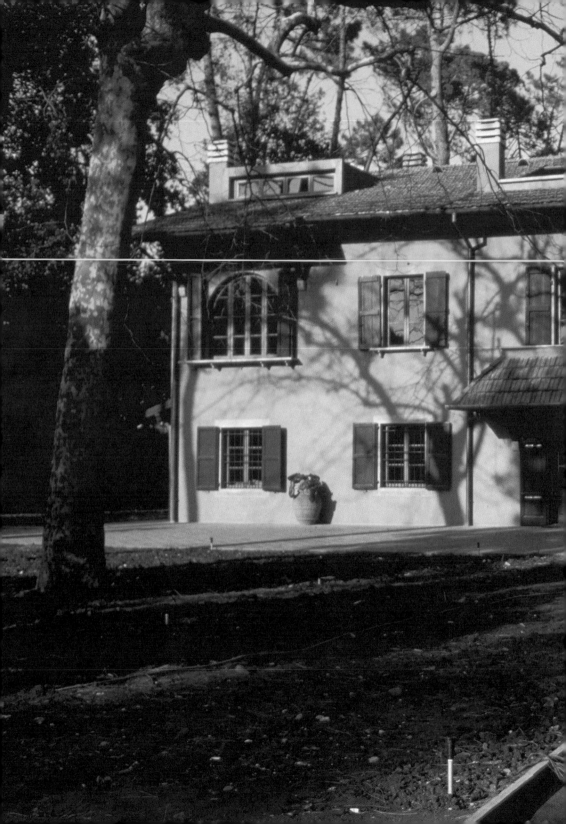

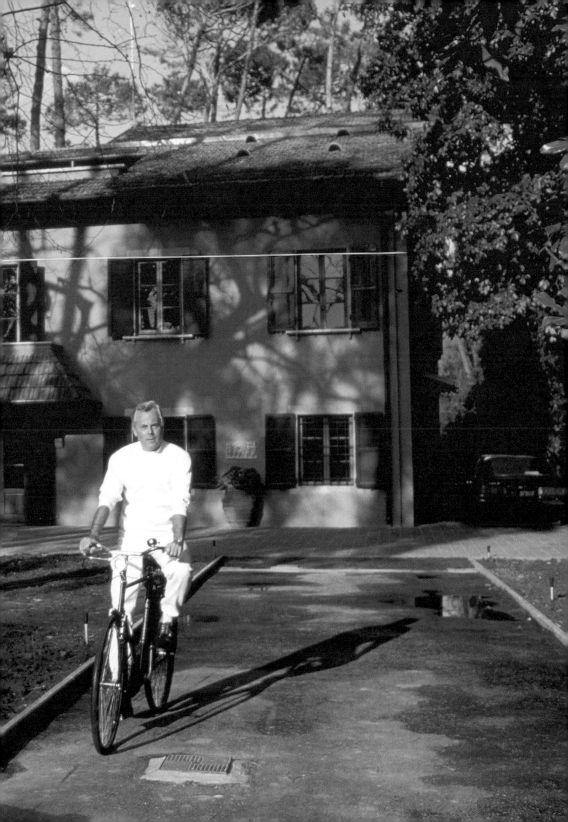

The fashion house of Armani is reported

to be the most financially successful that Italy has ever produced. Giorgio Armani first made fashion headlines in the mid-1970s, when he redefined the rules of tailoring by reinventing the jacket, making it far simpler. His name is known the world over and his eagle logo is instantly recognizable on a range of products that includes not only the main clothing ranges for men, women and children, but also jeans, skiwear, underwear, shoes, sunglasses, jewellery, hosiery, watches and perfume.

Yet in notable contrast to many of his fellow designers, Armani is notoriously reclusive; he keeps himself to himself, ostensibly shunning self-promotion and personal publicity. Unlike most other well-established fashion designers, there is relatively little published material devoted to Armani's work and no serious detailed analysis, other than of the cut and finish of his clothing designs. His garments do not grab the front pages through shocking or sensationalist designs, they are known for precisely the opposite – understated easy elegance. So why is the Armani label so successful?

Clues to the Armani enigma can be found in his early life. Born in Piacenza, 40 miles south of Milan, in 1934, Giorgio Armani is remembered as a sensitive and unusually fastidious child. Although he grew up in the years before and during the Second World War, he seems to have enjoyed a stable childhood. Armani describes his parents as middle-class, solid, hard-working people who were not wealthy but to whom "*fare bella figura*" (cutting a dash) was important. His mother was a vital influence on him in this regard, because, as Armani recalls, she dressed elegantly but disdained fashion. There are pictures of her on the Adriatic coast in the 1930s, holding young Giorgio's hand, looking streamlined and pared-down – uncannily like a model in an Armani advertisement. It is no surprise to learn that she favoured black, cream, white, taupe and grey.

G I O R G I O

Armani was the middle one of five children; one brother worked for the Milan department store La Rinascente while his sister Rosanna was a successful fashion model in the post-war years who worked, for example, for the leading Italian ready-to-wear company MaxMara in its early days. Hollywood films were a major form of entertainment in Italy in these years, and Armani consistently cites them as a lasting inspiration. His first impulse was to study medicine and even this, he says, was rooted in the idealism of film culture:

"THE **30S AND 40S** HAS ALWAYS **INFLUENCED ME**. THERE WAS AN elegant simplicity – CLEAN WHITE BLOUSE, A SIMPLE SKIRT, A DUSTER [COAT], A SLIM LAMÉ EVENING DRESS. BY THE **50s,** fashion WAS GETTING **TOO EXTREME**."

–*W*, FEBRUARY, 1991.

He told *Harpers & Queen* in October 1992 that: "I wanted to be a country doctor and save lives . . . like a hero in a Hollywood film."

However, his studies at the University of Bologna (from 1952) were interrupted by military service in 1953–54, including work in a military hospital, which extinguished both his idealism and his desire to continue his medical studies. In 1954 he took a job at La Rinascente, first as an assistant window dresser, then as an assistant fashion buyer, where he had an invaluable training in buying, in the use of fabrics and in marketing through customer profiling.

A R M A N I

In the 1960s, Armani joined Nino Cerutti's up-and-coming men's clothing company, where he worked for several years as a designer. Probably the most significant element of his work here was the development of his understanding of the industrial production of tailored garments and his increased appreciation of the value of fabrics in Italian fashion. The value lies in its technological experimentation, its adaptability and its willingness to create short production runs of special fabrics and to develop new textiles, especially luxury materials, such as the wools for which Armani became so well known.

This was precisely the period when the Italian fashion industry was consolidating the post-war success of its high-quality ready-to-wear sports- wear, made in fine, innovative fabrics, but before the extraordinary international explosion of Italian fashion, centred on Milan, in the 1970s. This was also when Armani met architecture student Sergio Galeotti, who became his intimate friend and with whom he launched his first own-label collection. In partnership with Galeotti, Armani successfully presented his first show under his own name at the age of 40, in 1974, in a Milan restaurant, to a handful of friends, buyers and journalists. According to the famous contemporary Italian fashion journalist Anna Piaggi, the first Armani collection made about £60,000 (*Vogue*, June 1979). His junior by 11 years, Galeotti was confident, ebullient and energetic and encouraged the establishment of the Giorgio Armani company the following year, with a reputed investment of £5,000.

Armani's great early innovation was his reconstruction of the traditional box-like man's jacket, by removing the lining, moving the buttons and the slope of the shoulders, in softer, lighter, unexpected fabrics that hung in a new way to form a more sensuous, comfortable and flattering garment that would suit both sexes. Initially, some fashion commentators pronounced that Armani's style was too low-key and asexual, but being on the periphery of fashion was just how Armani wanted to be perceived.

IN THE **1980s**, his suits BECAME THE **ULTIMATE** **"MUST-HAVE" SUBTLE** understatement.

Under Galeotti's shrewd management, the company expanded rapidly to become one of the outstanding business successes of the early 1980s, and the best-known Italian fashion label.

In 1981, the Emporio Armani chain was founded to sell to a younger market at around 60 per cent below the top Borgonuovo (or Black Label) line, and quickly became the backbone of the Armani empire. Today it is sold almost exclusively through Emporio stores at prices ranging from around £95 for a pair of jeans, to £250 for a beaded top, to £450 for a suit (against £1,100 for a Borgonuovo suit or £2,900 for an evening skirt). The garments are sold alongside a vast range of subsidiary products, with Emporio restaurants on hand to revive and encourage the flagging shopper.

THE FIRST FRAGRANCE OF MANY, **ARMANI LE PARFUM** WAS **LAUNCHED** IN 1982 AND IN THE SAME YEAR *Time* magazine made ARMANI THE FIRST **ITALIAN FASHION** DESIGNER TO APPEAR ON THEIR COVER, AND ONLY THE SECOND EVER FASHION DESIGNER, AFTER THE LEGENDARY Christian Dior.

In the late 1980s, the lower-priced womenswear range Mani (known as Le Collezioni in the US), was introduced, alongside Giorgio Armani Occhiali (glasses) and Giorgio Armani Calze (shoes).

These were followed in 1991 by the new A/X (Armani Exchange) line which was launched in the US in response to the economic recession. Inspired by the American PX stores, and described by some as "an up-market Gap", the range is considerably cheaper than the other clothing labels and is sold in specific Armani A/X boutiques, including a vast 10,000 square feet flagship store on Fifth Avenue, Manhattan. The strategy was successful and in the four years from 1994 to 1998 A/X sales quadrupled (*Women's Wear Daily*, September 8, 1998).

Armani describes his working method as "*disegno, tela, modificare*", (sketch, toile, modi-
fication); the key to the design process is in the translation from two to three dimensions,
from the page to the body. Production is industrialized, but in the top level collection there is,
he says, still some hand or "artisanal" work, which, he claims, is why his clothes are more
expensive than those of many of his rivals. This method helps him to achieve the standard of
fit and finish for which Armani is celebrated.

Galeotti's death in the mid-1980s was a great personal and professional blow. There
followed intense speculation about the future of the Armani company without its acknowl-
edged business-brain. As Armani told the *Sunday Times* in an interview on November 18, 1990,

"**SERGIO** protected ME
FROM EVERYTHING. **THE OUTSIDE**
WORLD WAS LIKE A FOREIGN COUNTRY TO
ME... **THEN HE DIED**... I HAD TO
defend myself FROM LAWYERS,
DEAL WITH THE **PRESS**, GET TO KNOW THE
people WHO WORKED FOR ME."

It took Armani a year to learn the business management of his company, and today he
manages to be both businessman and designer by dividing his time strictly between the two
areas. However, he continues to protect himself with those he trusts, such as his niece Silvana
(head of Emporio Armani), and still does not know most of the people who work for him. Most
of his team of young designers receive creative directives from intermediaries. "Mr Armani",
as he is always addressed, is now the sole owner and director of the company; his control is

absolute and extends to every facet of the empire.

"WORK IS MY life," ARMANI TOLD *HARPERS & QUEEN* IN OCTOBER 1992,
"I HAVE NO TIME FOR people."

Within the fashion industry he is almost as well known for his addiction to hard work and puritan personal habits, as he is for his designs. He is described as the most single-minded workaholic in the fashion business and his perfectionism is legendary. His personal appearance is always casual but impeccable, with neat grey hair and perhaps a navy cashmere sweater worn with a plain T-shirt and chinos. He neither drinks nor smokes and is said to have every piece of cutlery seal-wrapped. He professes to speak no English and leaves Italy infrequently. He has been described by the press over the years as diffident, secretive, shy, proud, obsessive, disciplined, immaculate and taciturn. Certainly, he is scrupulously discreet about his private life and keeps his impatience under control, most of the time. Control, it seems, is the key to understanding Armani's personality.

Staff must adhere strictly to a prescribed dress code (no nail polish and definitely no high heels). Even the distance between the hangers in his shops is dictated and carefully specified. For celebrity galas to launch new boutiques or ranges, he flies in the tablecloths and the silverware, not to mention the waiters' jackets. His models must walk the catwalk the Armani way – no sashaying, no hands-on-hips, no sexiness.

FOR ARMANI, "THE FASHION SHOW IS AN EXTREMELY serious THING" –*WOMEN'S WEAR DAILY*, OCTOBER 26, 1994.

He insists that the models wear white coats before the show, touches up their make-up himself and instructs them to "remember you are women, not young girls walking down the street . . . very elegant, very simple and very natural" (US *Vogue*, March 1992). He forbids them from applauding or making a lot of noise, and has earned his Milan presentation theatre the nickname of "the Church of Armani" among the fashion crowd. He avoids using star models because, he says, they intimidate his customers; it may also be because they are less keen to submit to the dictates of an Armani show.

By 1990 he had secured 23 licenses to design subsidiary products (typically made by diverse manufacturers in return for substantial royalties) for which he designed every item personally, instead of delegating the job as most big-name fashion designers do. Everything, from the packaging to the advertising campaigns, continues to be controlled directly by Armani himself. Yet as *Elle* magazine pointed out in July 1995,

"IT IS THIS fastidious ATTENTION TO DETAIL THAT ALLOWS AN ARMANI WEARER TO LOOK unstudied, UNDERSTATED AND, AT THE SAME TIME, perfect".

Armani's various homes have been created with the same attention to detail that pervades his business life. He owns a shuttered pink villa on the river Po (near his birthplace south of Milan), an English-style country house in the fashionable Tuscan seaside resort of Forte dei Marmi, a low-key house in St. Tropez, and, since 1998, a three-bedroom apartment on Central Park, with an enormous wraparound terrace, which he bought for a reputed $3 million, planning to spend four or five days there every other month. However, his best-loved home is a cement and glass retreat designed by local architect Gabriella Giuntolli on the remote volcanic island of Pantelleria between Sicily and the Tunisian coast, where he is said to keep a fleet of water-scooters for his guests. His days there are spent swimming, dining alfresco and watching films; he is reported to rent up to a hundred videocassettes before leaving Milan. All his homes are decorated in relaxed versions of the serene minimalist style that is so familiar to visitors to his stores, with wooden floors, neutral colours and pared-down furniture.

For years his company headquarters in Milan have been situated in a seventeenth-century palazzo on the elegant Via Borgonuovo. Original frescos and certain architectural details were screened off with beige panels when Armani moved in. His main apartment is on two floors at the centre of the palazzo; it is no surprise to learn that it is decorated in grey, white, beige and black, with smooth wooden floors, lit discreetly and furnished minimally with Jean-Michel Frank furniture and a few sculptures. In the basement is a one-lane swimming-pool and a theatre for fashion shows. In 1999, Armani converted an old chocolate factory on the outskirts of Milan into his new headquarters, to provide more than 129,000 square feet of offices and presentation space.

Armani's philosophy of style is not difficult to pinpoint: a synthesis of subtle, sophisticated, understated, minimal, languid and discreet modern elegance.

IT IS AN **ELEGANCE** THAT DOES NOT INVOLVE "dressing-up" AND IS **ABOVE ALL**, EASY-TO-WEAR; AS HE **HIMSELF** PUT IT: "I can't stand any kind of exhibitionism." *–ELLE*, MARCH 1993.

Armani chooses Michelle Pfeiffer as an example of someone who epitomizes his style: "She has an elegance, a simplicity, a purity of character. She really understands my clothes." (*Guardian*, May 29, 1994).

In Britain, the Armani name became practically generic in the 1980s, used to describe refined yet relaxed modernity in clothing, in muted colours. He softened men's clothing and fortified women's, bringing the sexes closer sartorially and easing the path towards late twentieth-century androgyny. He deconstructed the man's jacket and reconstructed it, without most of the structure and stiffening, on the more curvaceous lines of a woman's body, offering the successful working woman a synthesis of understatement and sensuality, femininity and power-dressing, without overexposure. Tailoring was combined with soft fabrics: chiffon skirts beneath sharp black jackets, for example. The beadwork for which he is renowned is simple in effect but often breathtaking in its craftsmanship, as seen, for example, on the bodices worn with "Scarlet O'Hara" skirts in spring/summer 1996. In fact, Armani sits on the border between what Rebecca Arnold, in her recent book *Fashion, Desire and Anxiety* (2000), identifies as "the seemingly contrasting values of luxury and restraint, reflecting in its balance between these elements of decadence and abstinence the fears and desires of contemporary culture".

Making the obvious contrast between the styles of Armani and his so-called "rival", the late Gianni Versace, Eric Clapton told US *Vogue* in March 1992 that

"Versace IS ALL ABOUT **SEX** AND **ROCK AND ROLL** – VERY RAUNCHY. Armani IS ABOUT **HARMONY**, HARMONY IN TONE AND COLOR AND FABRIC – HARMONY IN atmosphere."

Yet despite Armani's criticism of fashion designers who, he said, were turning fashion into "a porno show" through "the incarnation of low-level sexual fantasies" (*L' Espresso* magazine quoted in the *Sunday Times*, January 9, 1994), Armani's spring/summer 1994 collection showed unprecedented levels of "femininity", including bustiers and high heels for the first time. The designer explained this as a reflection of socio-economic change, expressing the belief that women no longer need to "dress like a man to be taken seriously" (*Women's Wear Daily*, October 26, 1994).

Armani acknowledges fashion but is not dominated by a need for novelty in every collection, and he deplores the flamboyance of several other Italian fashion designers. This is summed up in a rhetorical question asked of the US fashion trade paper *Women's Wear Daily* on October 26, 1994: "Should I continue down my own path or should I pick the path of the latest trend, the flashiest innovation? To show women in hotpants and skirts up to here?"

HIS CHANGES are never drastic, **RATHER,** HIS STYLES evolve OVER TIME.

His collections always include signature garments such as easy trouser suits and there are always muted colours present; any stylistic developments are typically presented towards the end of the show.

In September 1996, Armani caused a huge sensation in the international fashion press, when he was reported to have proclaimed that fashion was "dead" to the American weekly magazine *The New Yorker*. Versace retorted rather spitefully that "Giorgio thinks fashion is dead because he is no longer fashionable himself" (*Sunday Telegraph*, September 15, 1996). For his part, Armani protested:

"**I NEVER** SAID THAT. I SAID THE *diktats* OF fashion WERE DEAD. I MEANT THAT **WOMEN** HAVE LEARNT TO DRESS HOW THEY want. THEY WON'T BE DICTATED TO BY **ONE DESIGNER** ANY MORE." *–SUNDAY TELEGRAPH*, MARCH 9, 1997.

Despite the thematic continuity of understatement and languid androgyny in his designs, Armani's style has in fact seen several revolutions in his company's quarter-century. The line was founded with the unconstructed jacket, with sloping shoulders, narrow lapels, baggy pockets and loose weave fabrics that draped on both men and women. At the end of the 1970s, Armani lowered the neck, extended and padded the shoulders and widened the lapels to create the famous wedge-shaped power-suit. In the mid-1980s he abandoned the power-suit for the roomier "sack-suit". In the light of his 1994 denunciation of hotpants, it is interesting to see that Armani's spring/summer collections for 2000 included sequinned hotpants.

Armani's overriding quest in clothing style seems to have been to change attitudes to dressing, to change ideas about what is and what is not acceptable. He has played with Eastern fabrics in Western styles and Western fabrics in Eastern styles; spring/summer 1994 was an important collection which drew heavily on North African themes for simple trouser suits with soft jackets, and loose jellaba overshirts with slim pyjama-style trousers, all in the highest-quality Italian fabrics.

HE HAS ALSO MADE AN IMPORTANT contribution TO LATE twentieth-century FASHION HISTORY BY USING FABRICS traditionally ASSOCIATED WITH MENSWEAR FOR WOMEN, AND VICE VERSA.

Armani faces more competition these days, particularly in the menswear field, but is happy, he says, that there is a lot more variation and that men can dress in Ralph Lauren, Versace or Armani, according to their personality, rather than being confined to one traditional look. He is especially happy that "Eric Clapton can wear a collarless shirt with a suit and it is considered elegant. It has taken twenty years to achieve that." (*GQ*, March 1994).

Armani professes to abhor the Versace approach to marketing and says he would never use a show business personality in an advertising campaign, as Versace did, for example, with Madonna. Yet for all his protestations, Giorgio Armani has developed a hugely significant relationship with the movie and rock industries, reflecting his self-confessed "movieholism". Armani's style has been promoted by various Hollywood stars for many years, both on screen and off – from Richard Gere, lounging in a cream Armani suit, trying to seduce Lauren Hutton in *American Gigolo* in 1980, and Sean Connery, Kevin Costner and Robert de Niro in *The Untouchables* (1987) to Harrison Ford, Michael Douglas, Tom Cruise, Nicole Kidman, Sharon Stone and Winona Ryder, who have all worn his designs at high-profile events.

Armani was reputedly the first fashion designer to employ a full-time Los Angeles repre-sentative to woo actors into wearing his clothes on public occasions. In 1991, Cindy Crawford and Richard Gere were married in complementary Armani suits. Michelle Pfeiffer wearing a plain dark trouser suit to the Oscars was an influential moment in fashion history as well as in the history of the Academy Awards, and at the 1995 Oscars, Jodie Foster and Annette Bening both wore beaded Armani gowns, all reported widely in the international press.

From the late 1980s, Armani has capitalized on his links with the stars and staged a series of all-star events. One of the most celebrated was the premiere of his film auto-biography, *Made in Milan*, which he commissioned from director Martin Scorcese, at the Venice Film Festival in 1990, which was attended by a strategic selection of big names, such as Meg Ryan and Uma Thurman and once again made headlines in the world's fashion press. The theme of the film is that Armani's life (or at least the one he reveals), is an intrinsic part of his work – Armani's lifestyle is a reflection of his design aesthetic.

Interestingly, his clothes are generally worn by well-established names, such as Jodie Foster, Isabella Rossellini, Julia Roberts and now Gwyneth Paltrow, rather than by those on the way up who need to make a splash in the world's press. For such established stars his elegant, simple clothes provide a good foil. As Donald Sutherland told US *Vogue* in March 1992:

" WEARING Armani IN HOLLYWOOD MAKES NO STATEMENT, IT MAKES YOU LOOK AS individual AND terrific AS POSSIBLE ".

Although Armani is better known for film clothing, he has made a few sorties into other areas of the performing arts. In 1994, Jonathan Miller, one of Britain's most illustrious opera directors, commissioned Armani to dress the cast of his 1995 production of *Cosi Fan Tutte* at Covent Garden. This was Armani's first major effort on stage. The set could have been one of the designer's own homes, with its blank walls and simple floor cushions. The clothes were mostly chosen off-the-rack from Armani's current Emporio collections. The male "lovers" wear Armani suits throughout, but for the final scene the two main female characters appear in wedding dresses adapted from evening gowns in the Giorgio Armani collection; covered in tulle veils, they glisten in sparkling beaded dresses. The Armani connection was covered by broadsheet newspapers in both Europe and the US and served to underline Armani's reputation as a designer for the erudite.

More recently, in 1996, Armani famously designed the costumes for Joaquin Cortés's sensational "flamenco-fusion" dance spectacular which took Europe by storm. Not surprisingly, the costumes were not clichés of Spanish traditional dance costume, with swirling capes, matador jackets and ruffles, but simple, sinuous, sensual and easy to move in, in plain colours. The enormous international publicity that surrounded the production offered excellent publicity for Armani.

In 1990 the US accounted for approximately one-third of Armani's total annual turnover, making him the biggest-selling European fashion designer in the US (*Sunday Times*, November 18, 1990). Today, Armani is a billionaire. In 1999, the company's retail network included 53 Giorgio Armani stores, 6 Le Collezioni stores, 129 Emporio Armani, 48 A/X Armani Exchange stores, 4 Armani Jeans and 2 Armani Junior stores in 33 countries. In 1999, the company acquired property on Milan's Via Manzioni, intended to house new Emporio Armani and Armani Jeans outlets, alongside the first Armani Casa (housewares) store, stocking an entirely new range of products, from furniture to bedlinen, and two restaurants; this complex is due to open in Autumn 2000.

Even as he speaks of retiring, Armani continues to clamour for further global growth, and has made a significant decision to modernize the style and image of his company. He is looking for a dramatic change in vision. This vision encompasses the entire style and image of the Armani label, from clothing design through to advertising. At the end of the 1990s, Armani deliberately moved away from the traditional cool nonchalance of black-and-white promotional images which reinforced his stylistic ideals, by photographers such as Peter Lindbergh, known for his understated precision. Instead he brought in Ellen Von Unwerth, to introduce colourful sexuality, and to "give the pictures a modern attitude". As he told Colin McDowell in 1999:

"IT WAS time FOR A CHANGE. I WANTED IMAGES THAT REFLECTED young minds AND A MODERN WAY OF BEING."

–*SUNDAY TIMES*, JULY 25, 1999.

This new promotional approach reflected an important change of direction in Armani's design studios. Armani decreed that although he wanted to preserve the sophisticated slim elegance of his style, he sought a more youthful, colourful look; although he wanted to build upon his reputation for beautiful beadwork, he wanted to develop it in a more trendy way. The spring/summer 1999 collections revealed a new sportiness alongside the expected understated jackets, in response to the popularity of "ulitity chic". The main line surprised with shocking pink and rich, radiant orange for evening wear. Anyone who thinks that Armani is only about beige suits need look no further than the spring/summer 2000 collections. Alongside the usual neutral jackets and trousers was an unexpected confection of pastel shades mixed with bolder colours (including hot pink suede and rainbow-striped swimwear), together with funky sequins and pixie boots.

In July 1999, Armani released solid sales figures for the previous year. Although Giorgio Armani SpA disclosed figures for previous years, this report was far more detailed than usual, and was designed to bolster the aspirations of the designer, who believes, as he told *Women's Wear Daily*, that his "golden moment is yet to come" (*Women's Wear Daily*, August 2, 1999). In particular, Armani is thirsting for an increased share of the US market. The US now equals Europe (excluding Italy), at 33 per cent of the total turnover, with Italy at 18 per cent, Japan at 7 per cent and the rest of the world at 9 per cent.

The report showed that net income grew over 10 per cent to $134 million in 1998 and that retail turnover had increased by a similar level to an impressive $3.28 billion. It is particularly significant that this reflected fervent efforts to expand fragrance and accessory sales and that the company was keen to go much further in this direction in the twenty-first century. This is presumably because clothing sales are a falling percentage of the total Armani turnover, at 58 per cent in 1998, against 63 per cent in 1997, (with womenswear accounting for just over half of this), while fragrances rose to a massive 42 per cent (from 37 per cent) in the same period.

In July 1999 Armani cemented his quest for modernization with the appointment of a new creative director, Matthias Vriens, 36, editor of avant-garde Paris magazine *Dutch*. Vriens not only heads the creative studio, but is also responsible for overseeing advertising campaigns, packaging design, retail merchandising concepts and special events. Through this appointment, and the selection of a new team of US executives, the company is trying to "create an infrastructure that is more compatible with the way business is done in the US", as

Andrew Grossman, of Giorgio Armani US, explained to *Women's Wear Daily* on August 2, 1999.

Armani has no obvious heir and it is well known that he is mulling over a joint venture with, or perhaps a take-over by, another fashion group. In May 1999, Armani told *Women's Wear Daily* of his admiration for Bernard Arnault, the acquisition-hungry head of LVMH (Louis Vuitton Moët Hennessy), and suggested him as a possible joint-venture partner. There has, however, been no confirmation of any formal agreement from either party.

Like all other successful fashion designers, Armani is selling a seductive illusion.

Armani's glamour comes through association, with hand-picked, impeccably presented staff, evocative advertising campaigns and the celebrities he cultivates.

ONE OF THE KEYS TO Armani's success HAS BEEN HIS UNDERSTANDING OF CHANGING SOCIO-ECONOMIC MOOD.

His success cannot be attributed to one single factor, but to a timely blend of factors. He understood back in the mid-1970s, that although consumers were rejecting formality in favour of more casual clothing, they did not want to give up elegance. He also recognized the shift in the socio-economic position of women and reflected the change in gender relations by bringing womenswear closer to men's and vice versa. In the early to mid-1980s, he benefited from the need to express power and status through clothes, and from the late 1980s his minimal style has attracted those who wished to be seen as cultured or serious. The Armani look continues to represent a key strand in Italian fashion style.

Furthermore, it should not be forgotten that he was extremely fortunate in his choice of business partner in Sergio Galeotti, whose incisive dealings allowed him to focus on design in the formative years of his company. His appreciation of, and access to, the Italian textiles industry was also fundamental to his success. Lastly, the extent of control that Armani has maintained throughout his empire and his attention to detail, ensure that he has not become complacent and is always searching for expansion and improvement.

Although today, he has given over most of his headlines to the likes of Prada and Gucci, his products continue to sell extraordinarily well, largely because there remains a significant proportion of the population that is most comfortable in elegantly understated clothes and accessories and enjoys a balance between tradition and modernity. Clearly, there are still plenty of Armani customers, especially in America, but on the whole they are not getting any younger;

IT WILL BE **FASCINATING** TO SEE WHETHER Armani's recent EFFORTS TO **REJUVENATE** THE ARMANI IMAGE AND TO **REORGANIZE** THE COMPANY ARE **SUCCESSFUL** in the long term, AND INDEED WHETHER IT WILL **FLOURISH** OR FAIL, WHEN HE FINALLY RELINQUISHES **TOTAL CONTROL.**

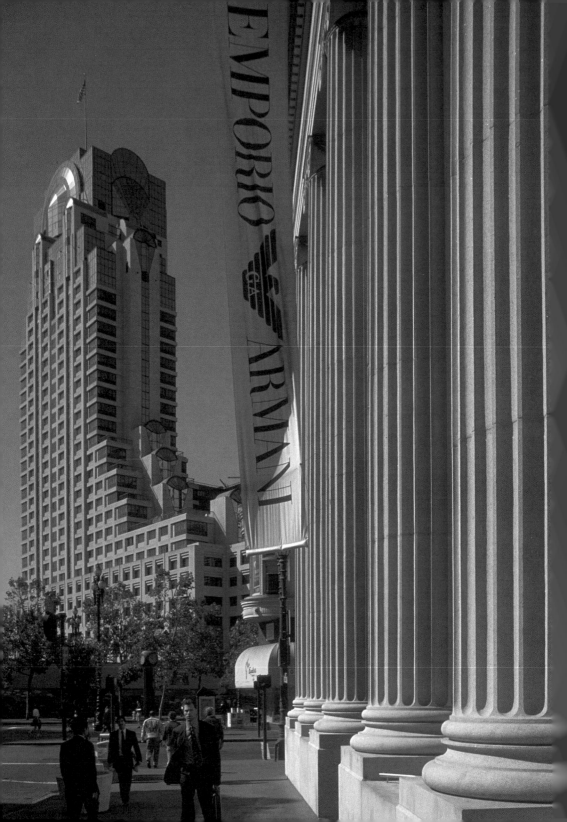

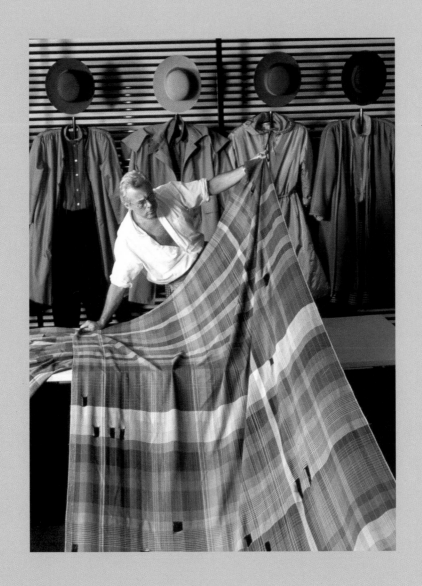

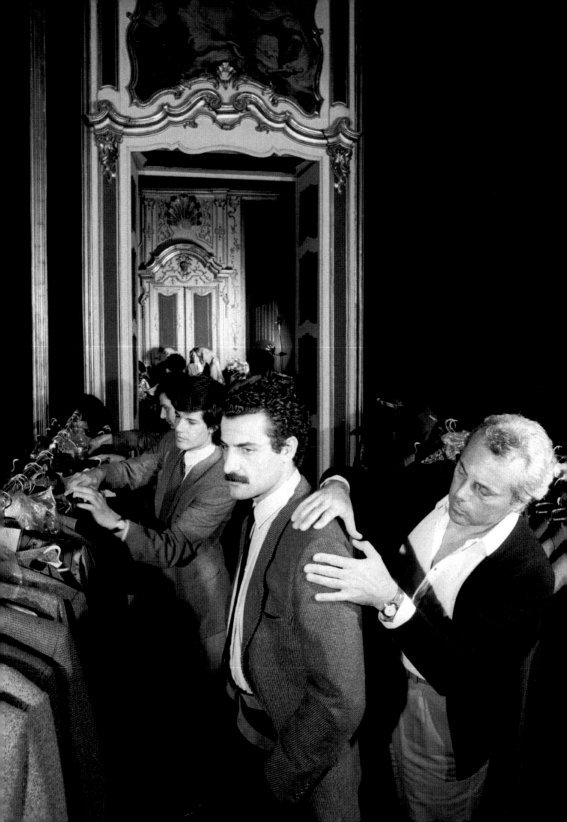

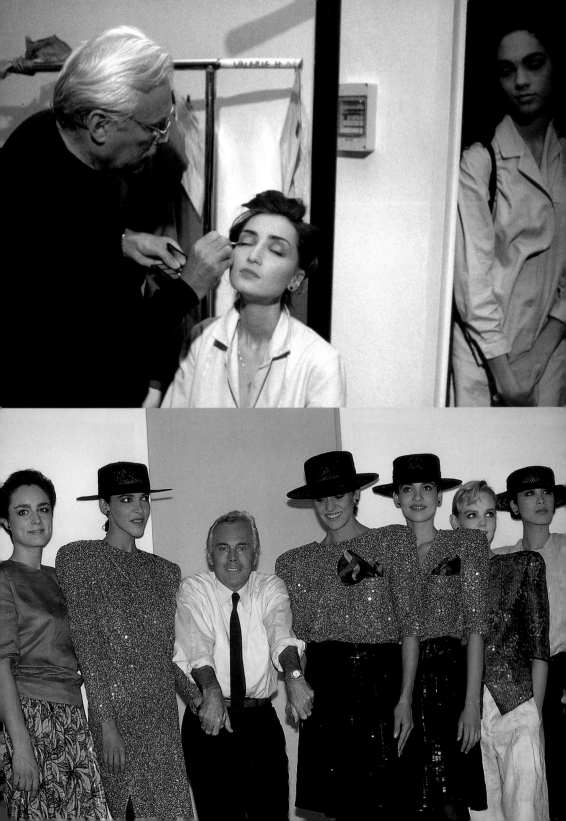

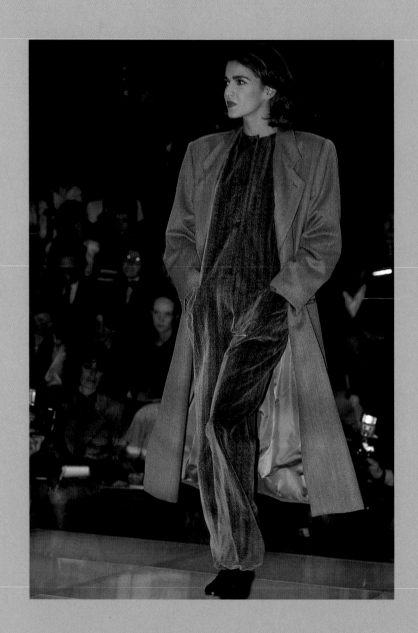

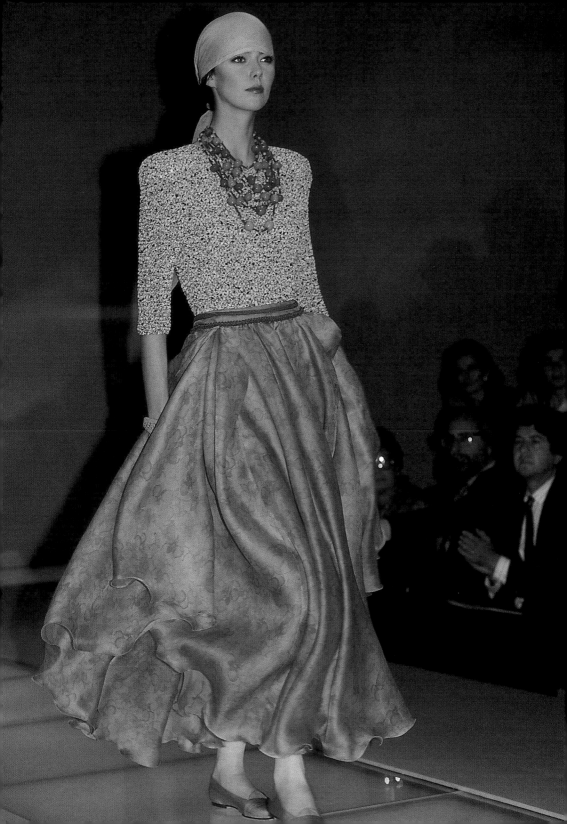

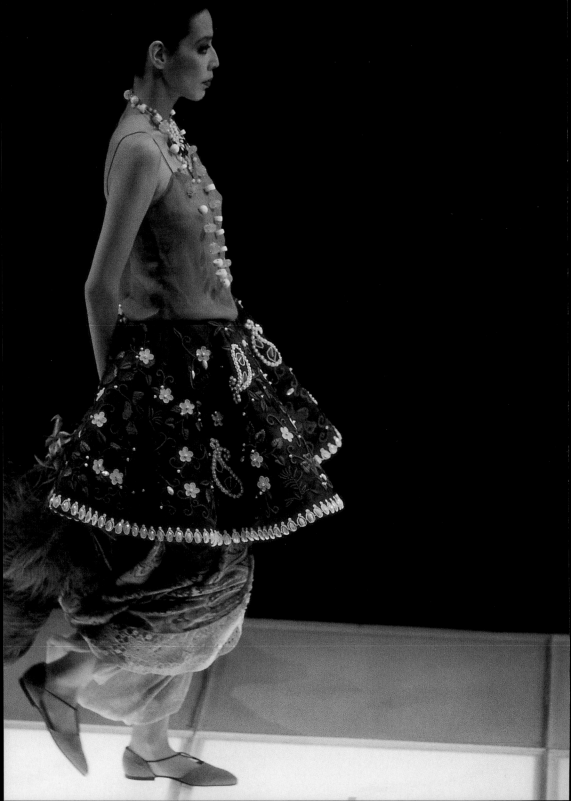

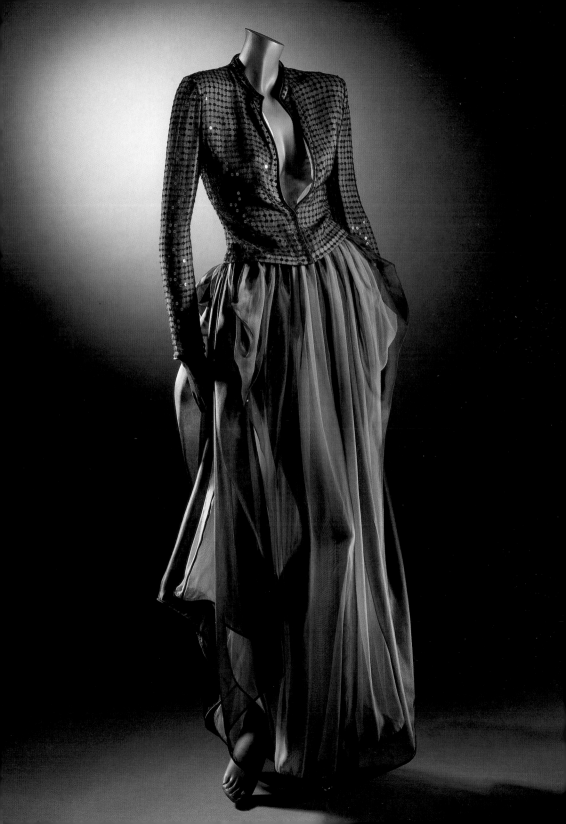

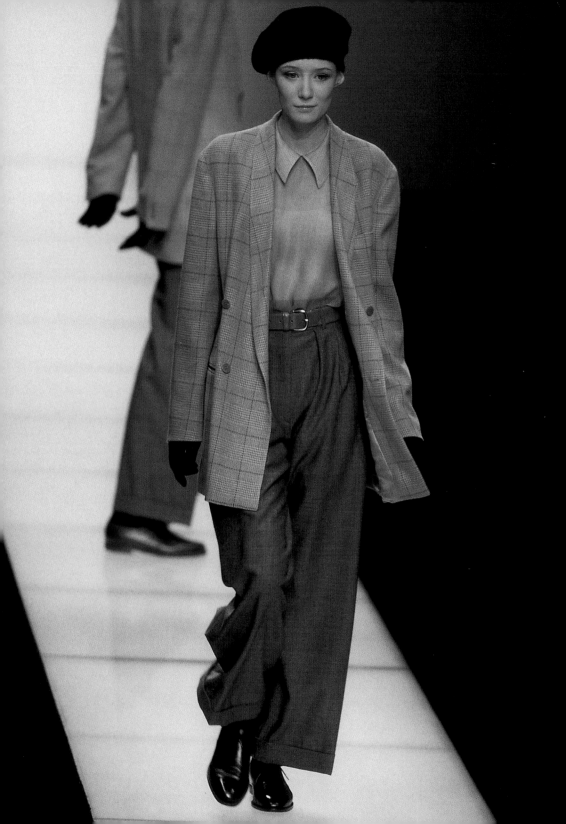

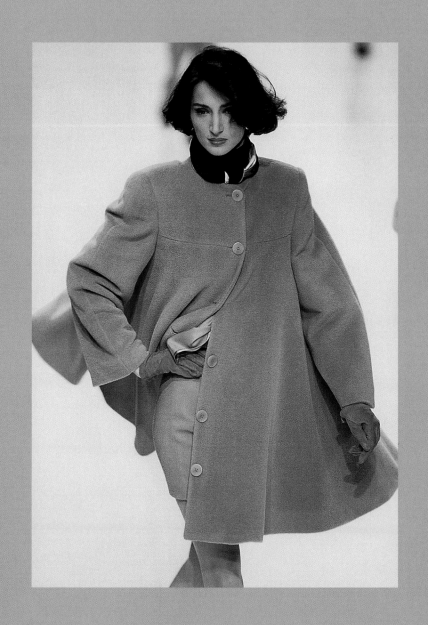

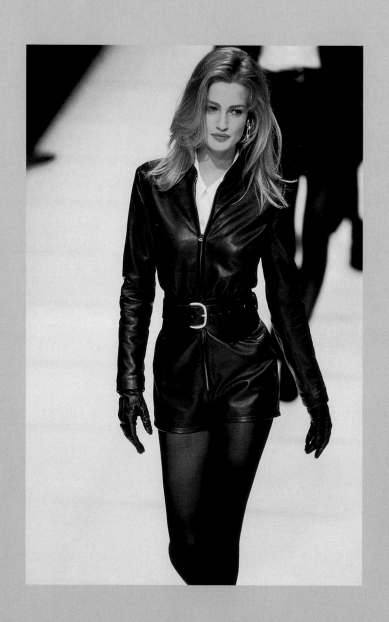

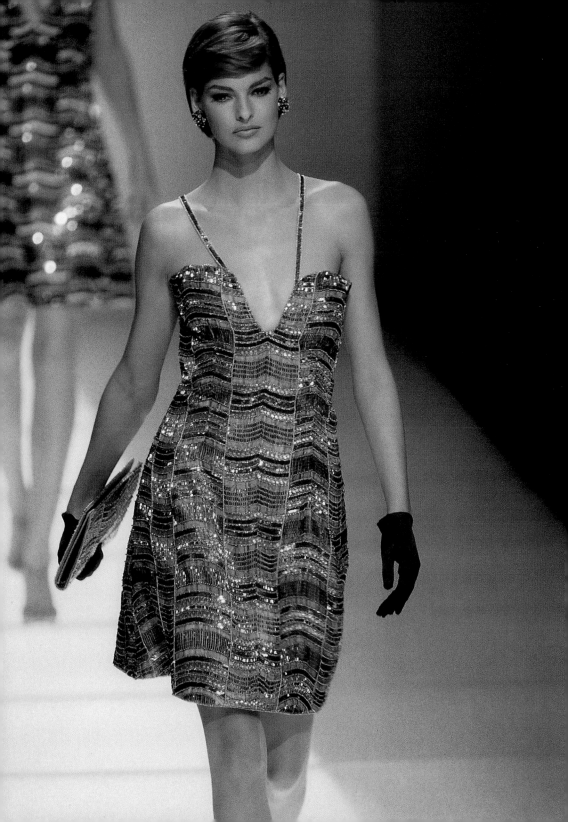

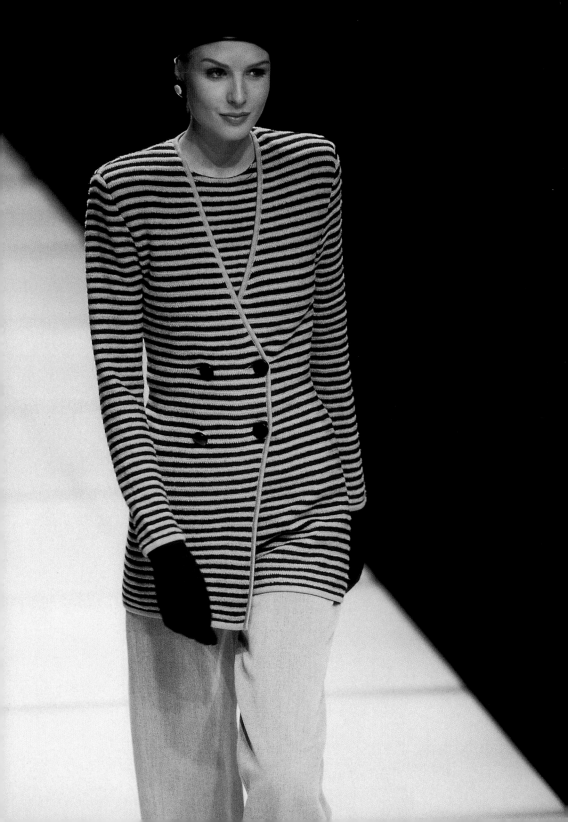

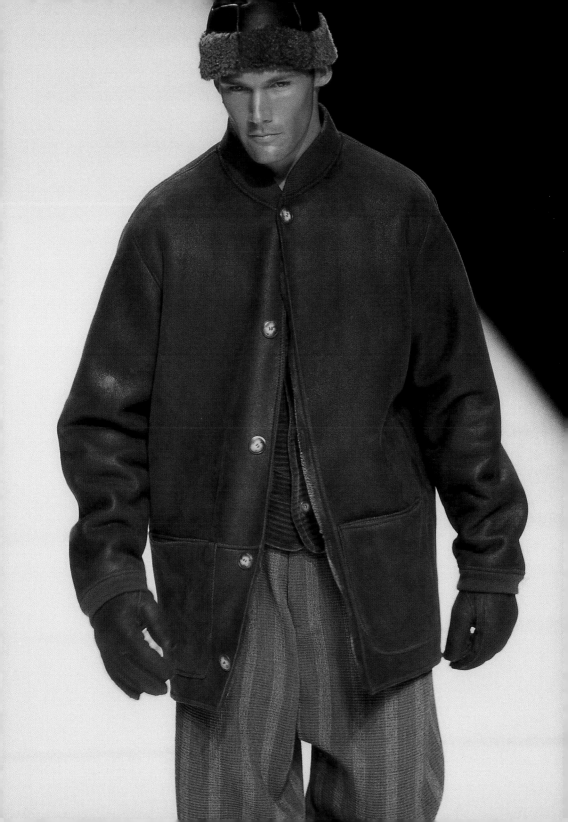

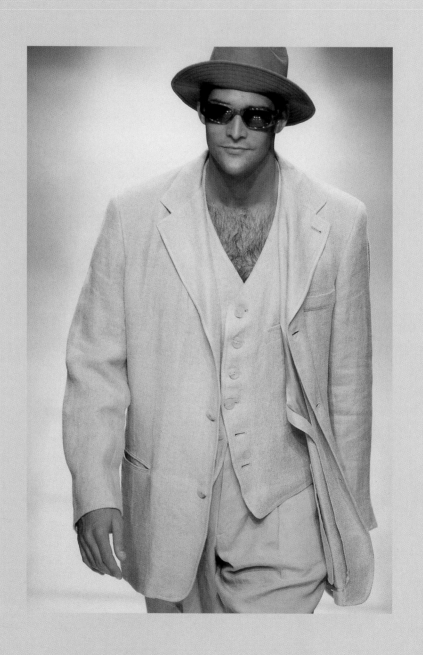

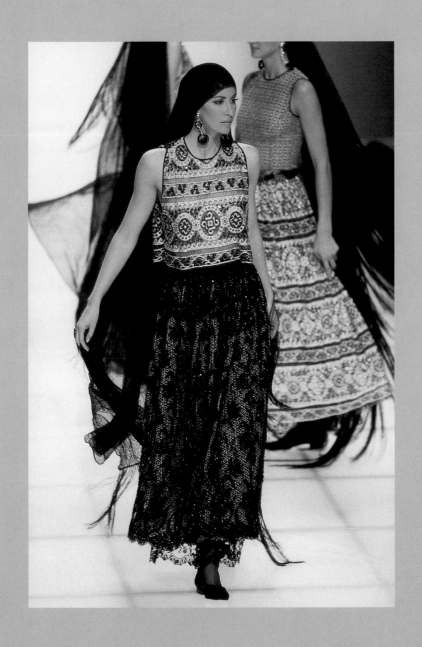

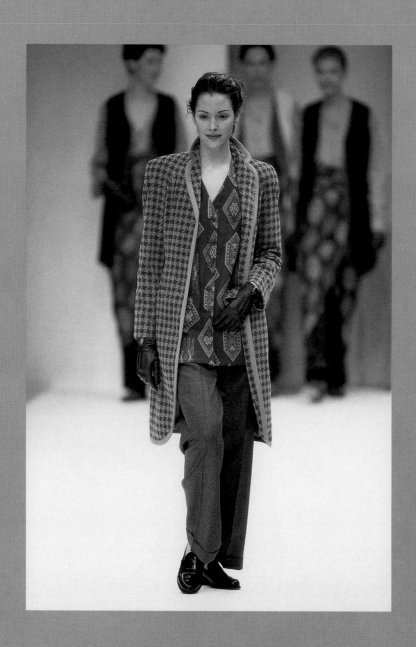

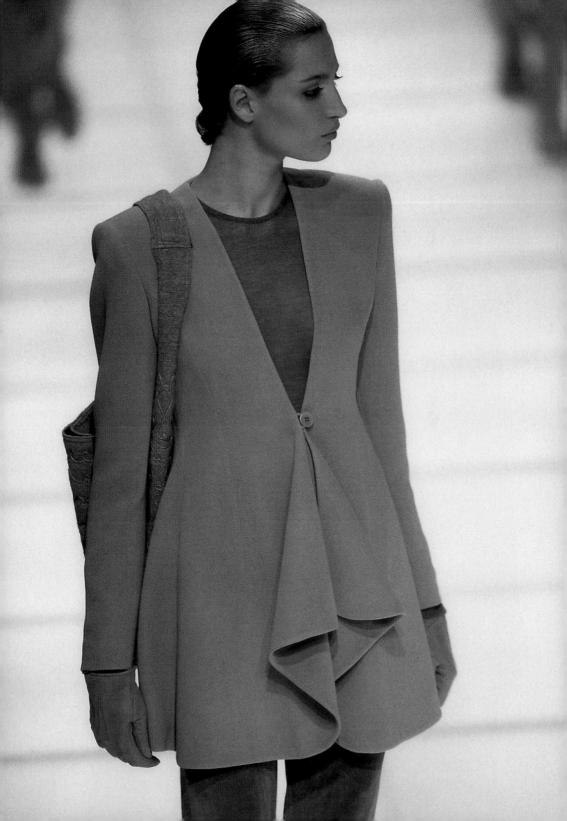

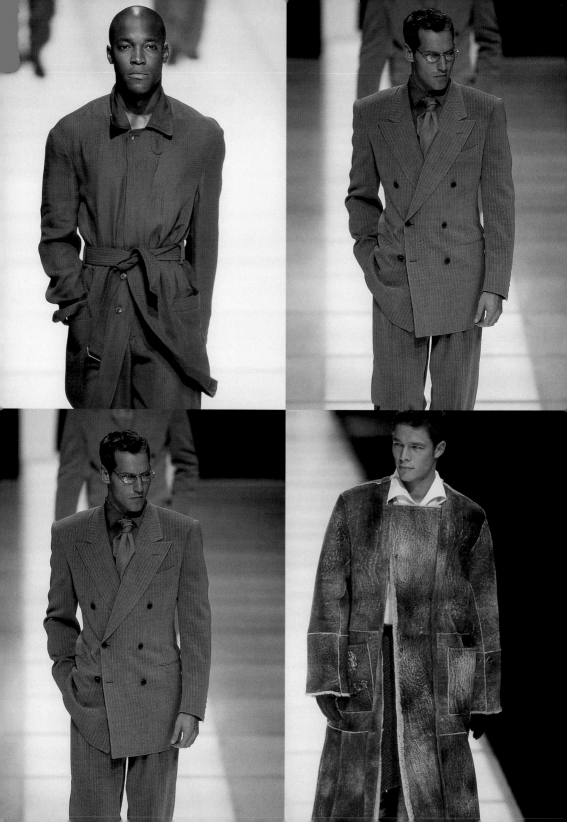

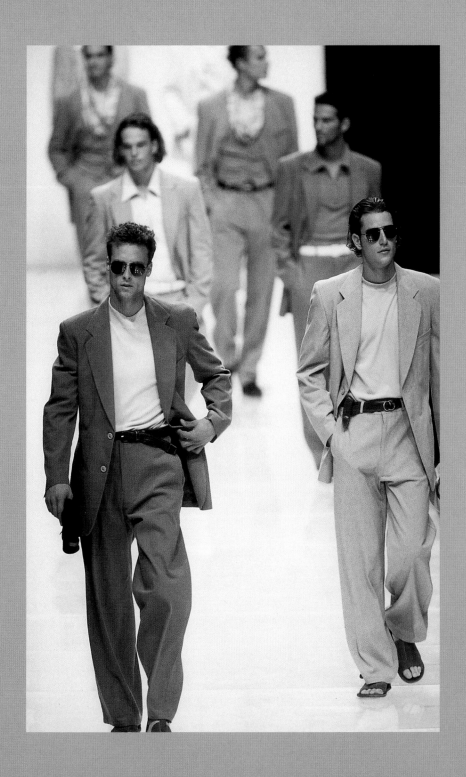

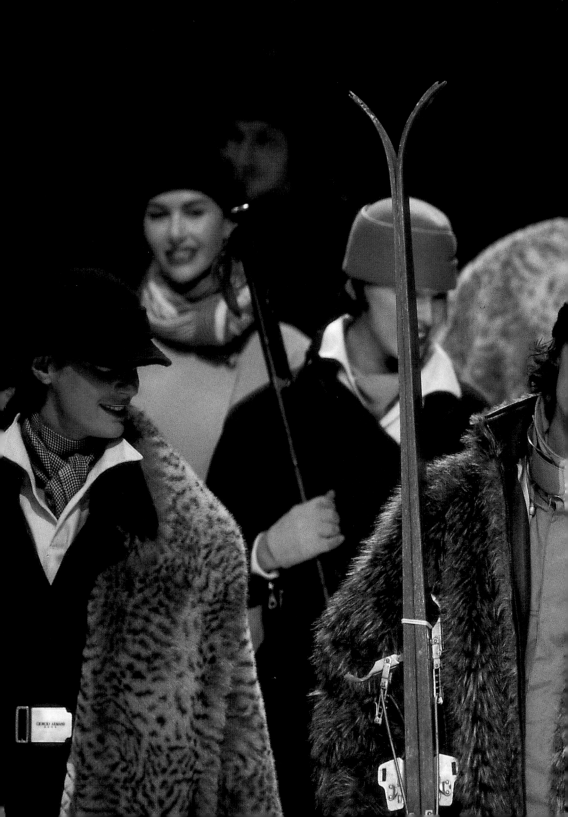

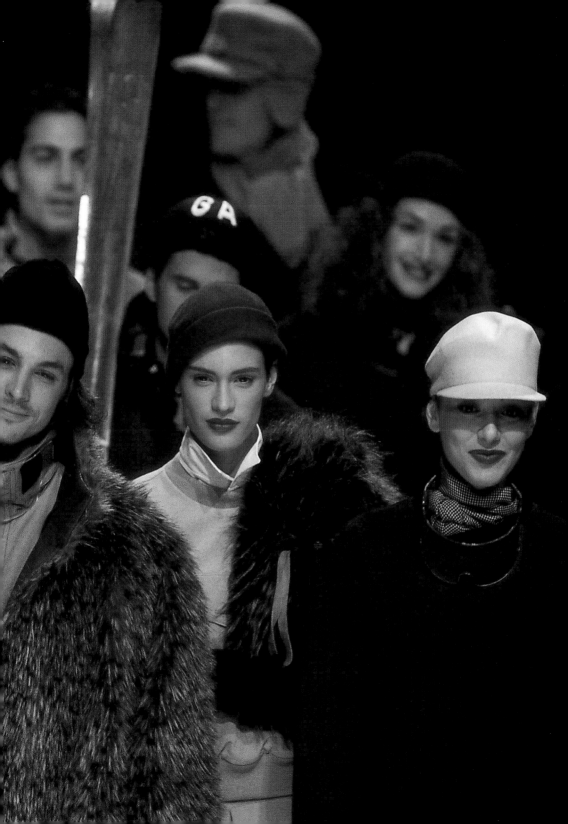

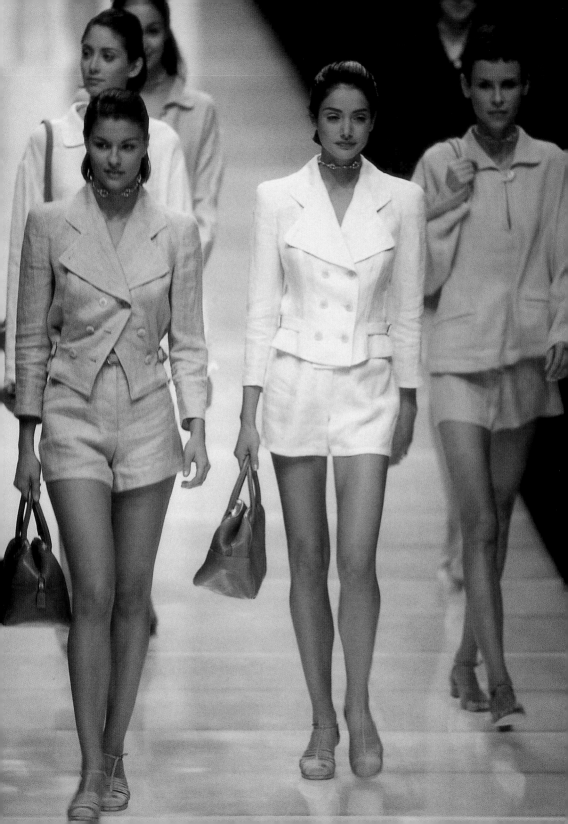

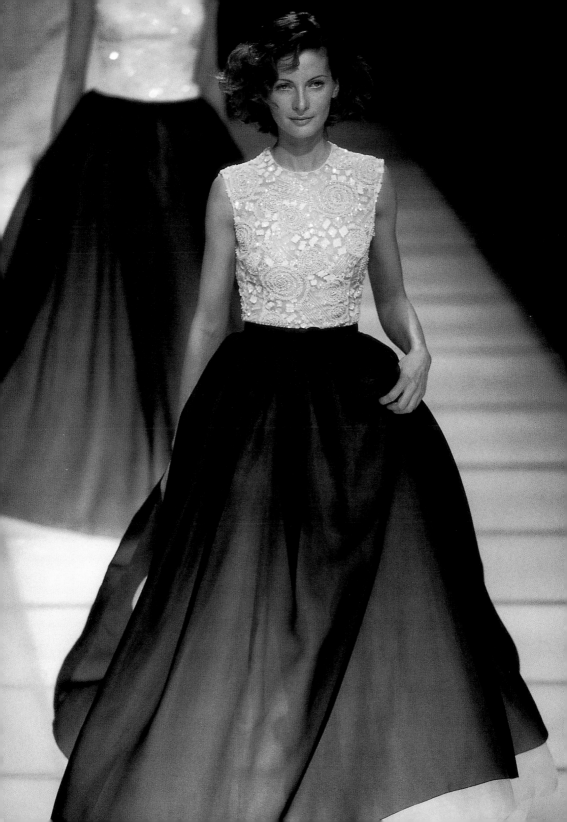

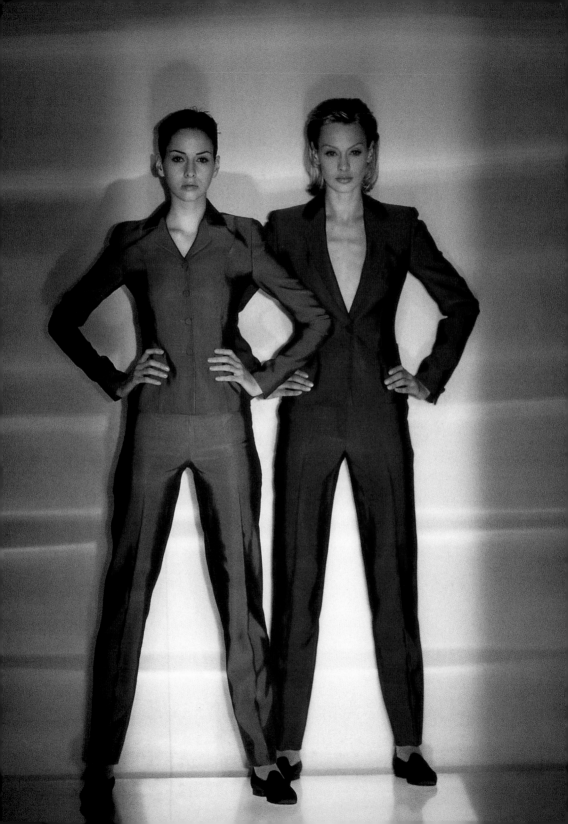

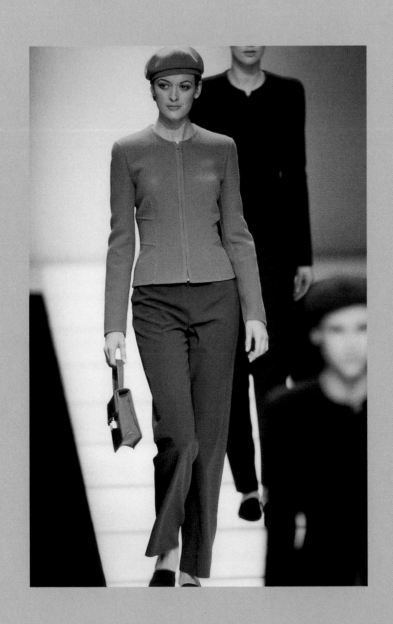

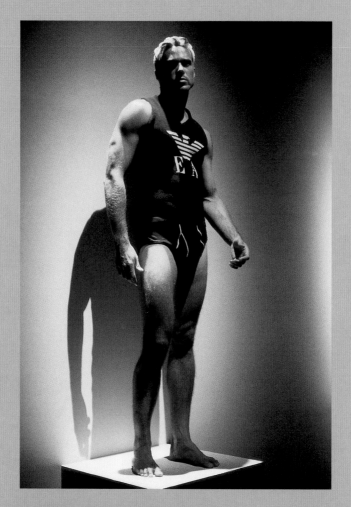

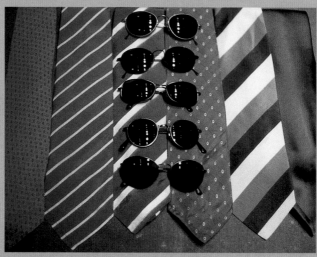

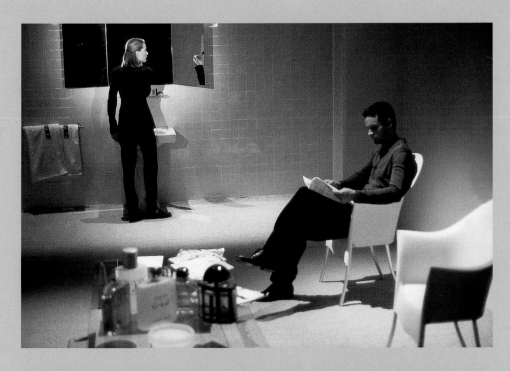

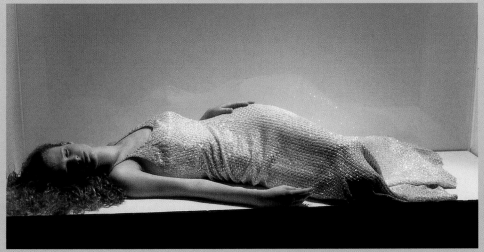

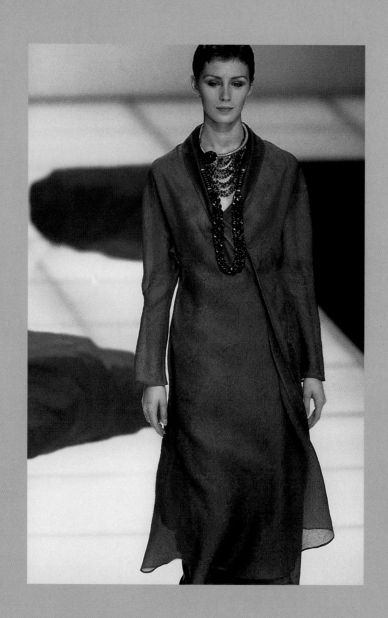

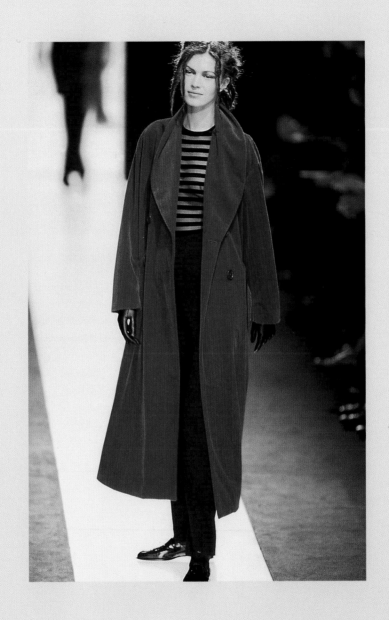

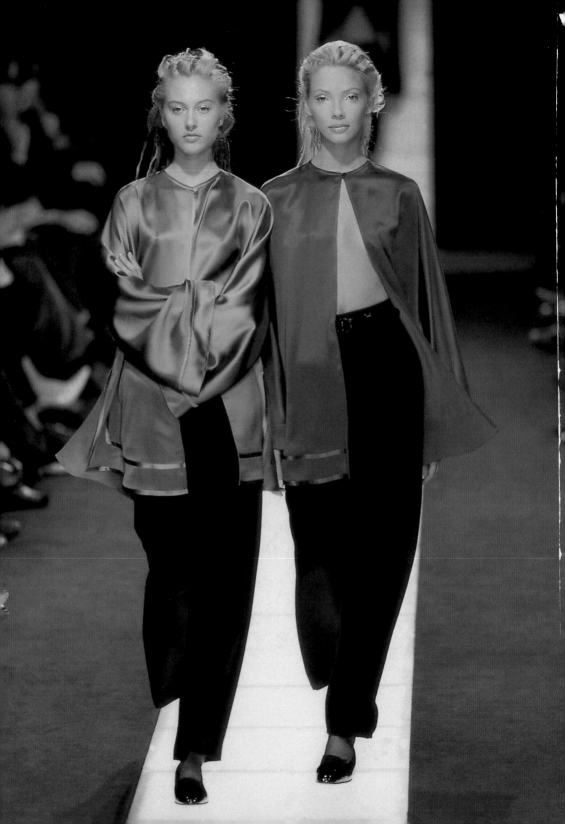

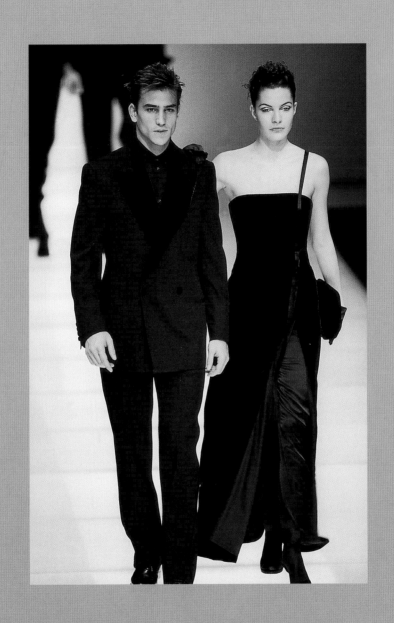

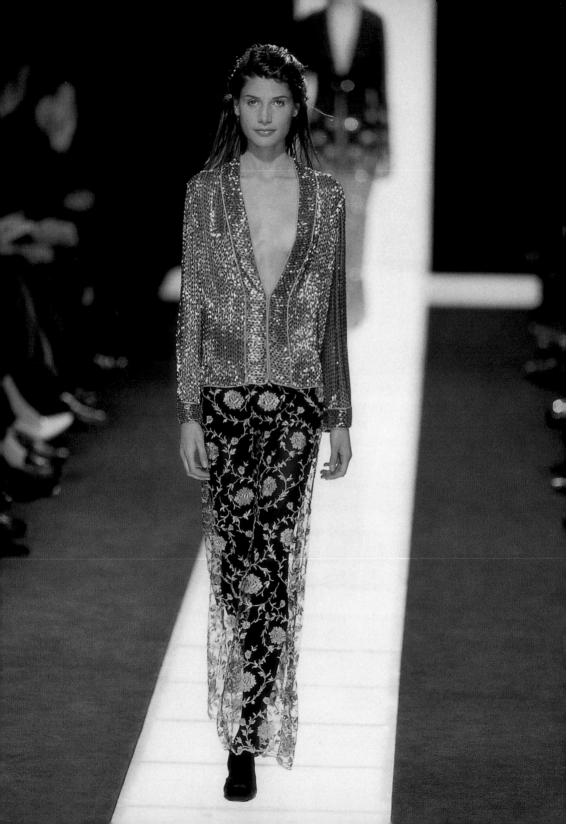

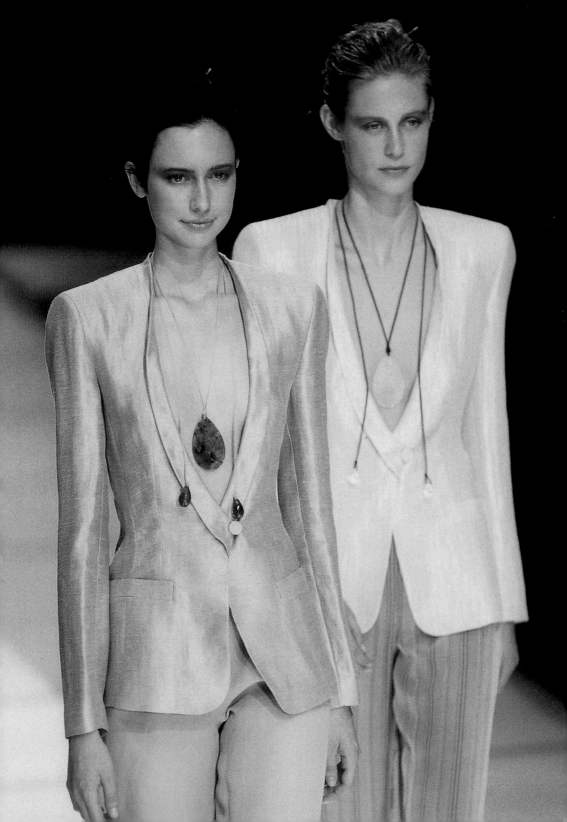

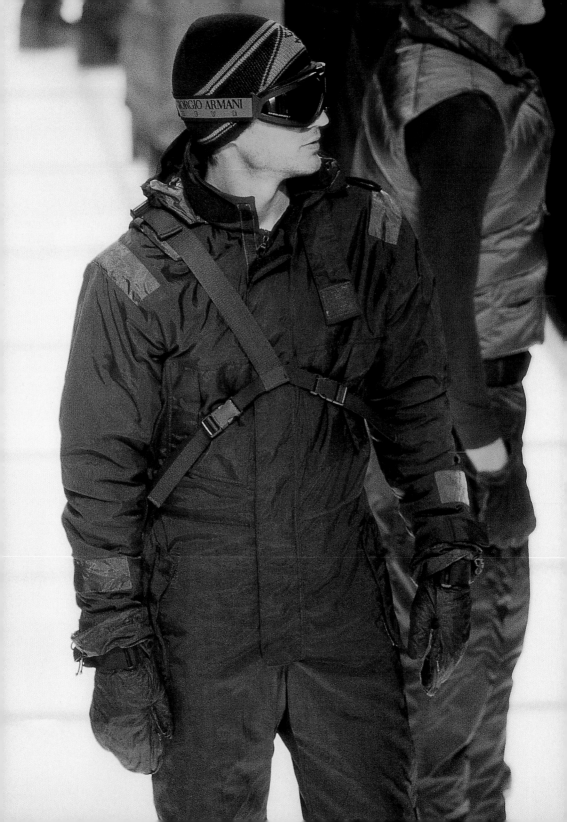

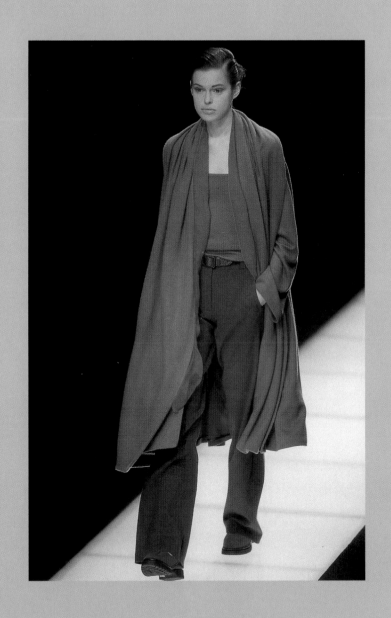

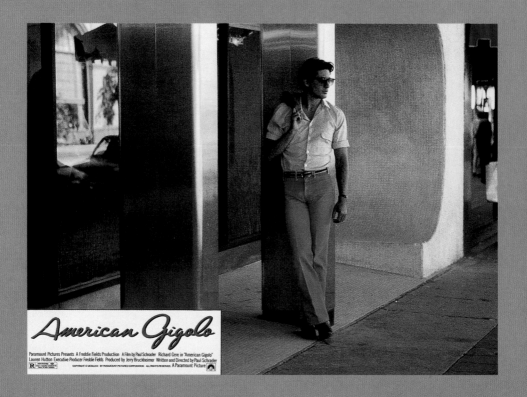

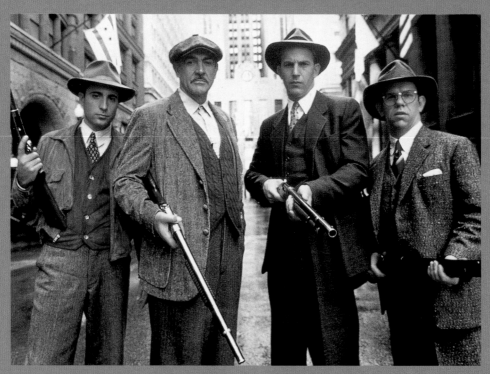

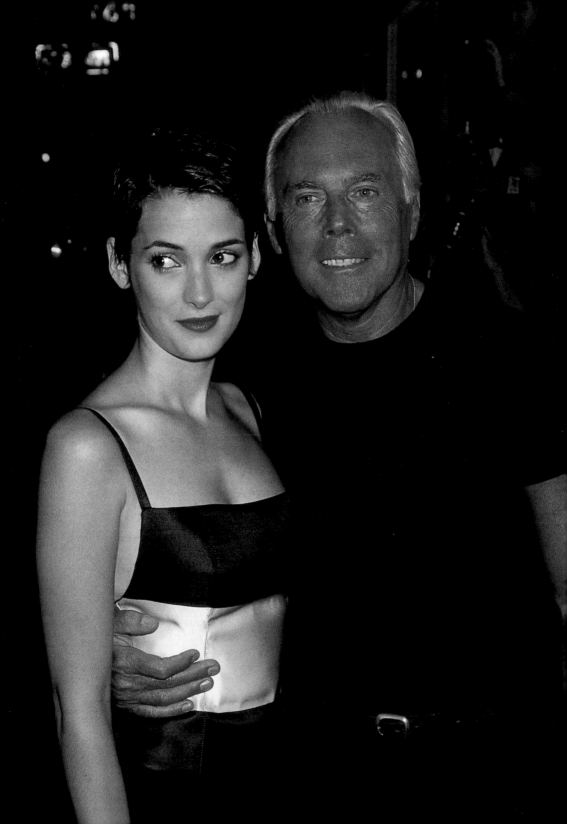

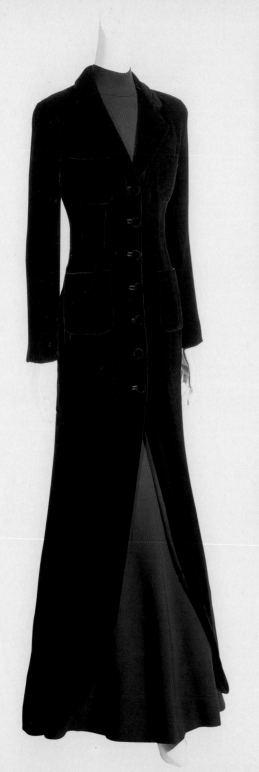
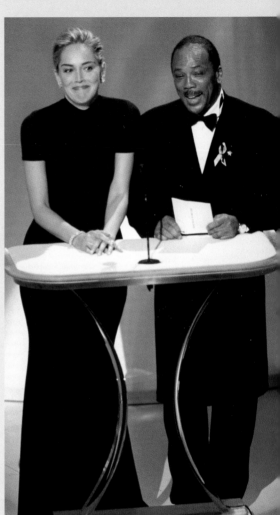

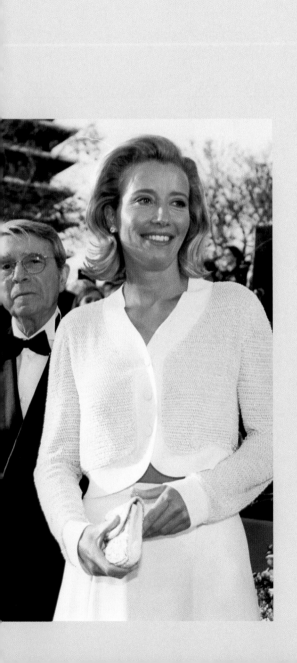
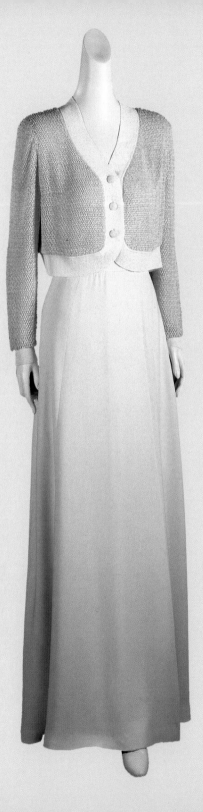

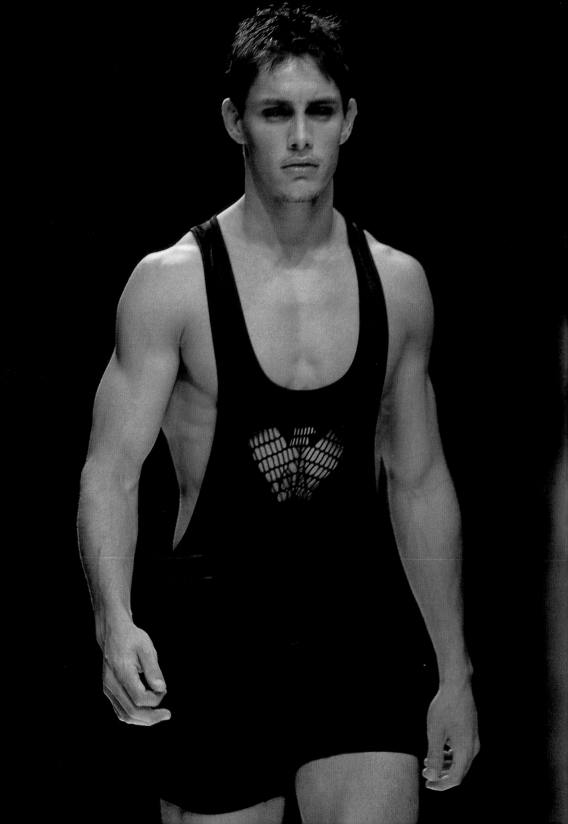

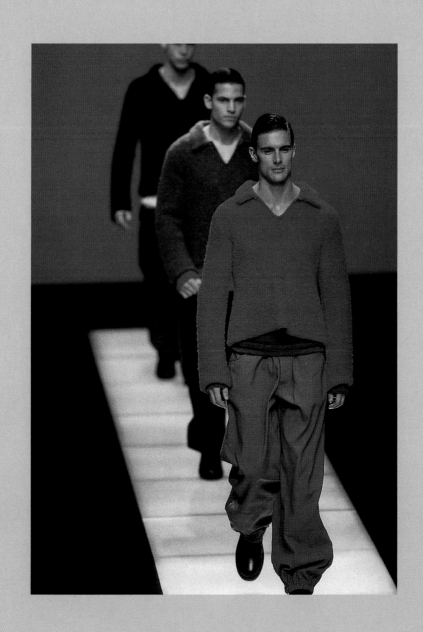

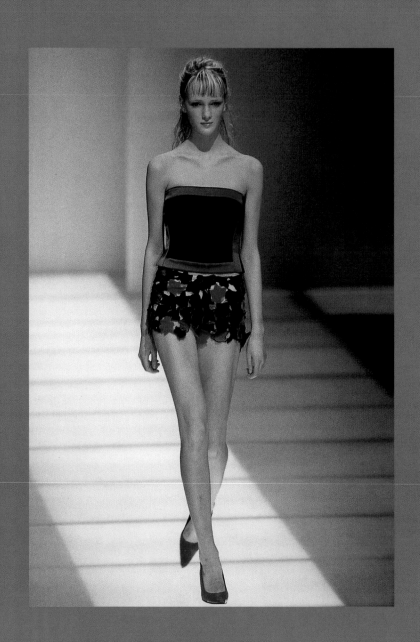

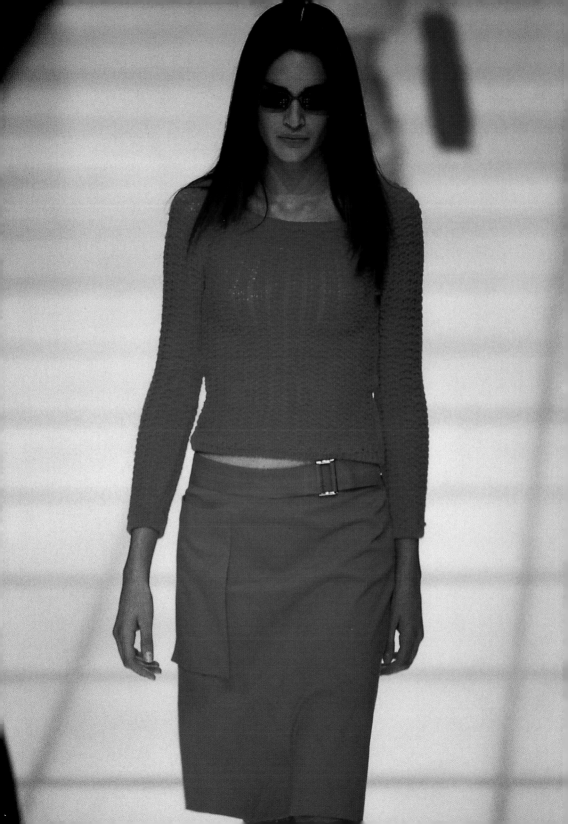

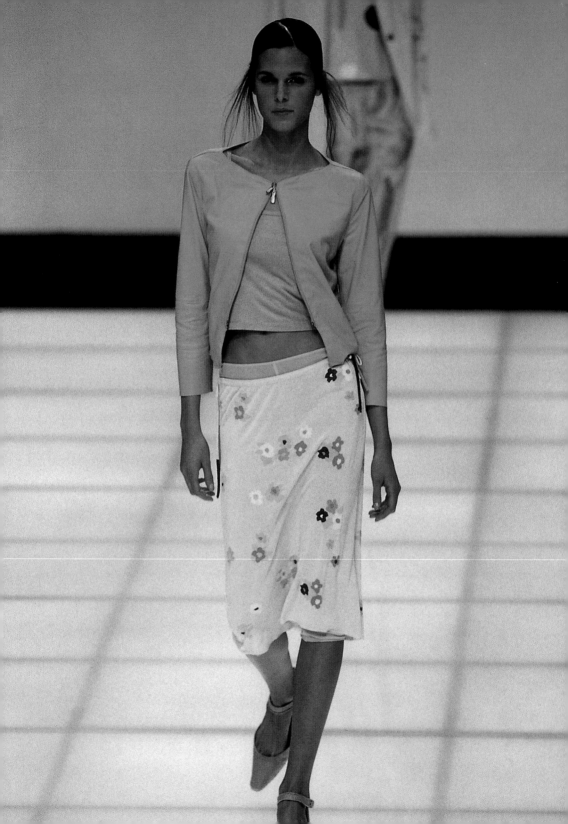

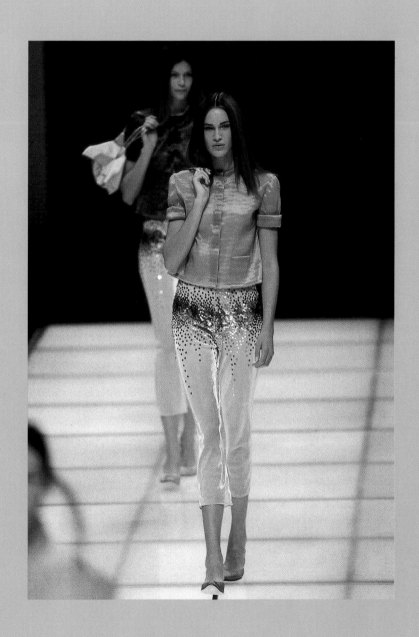

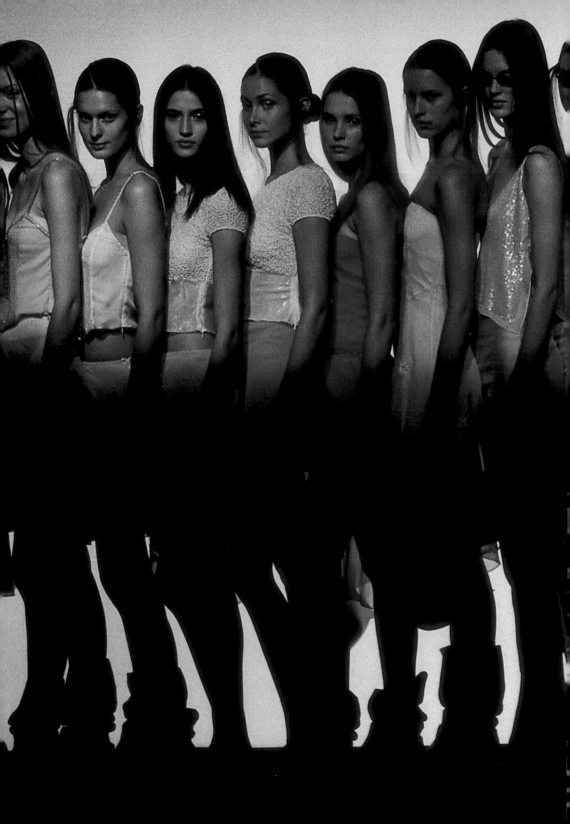

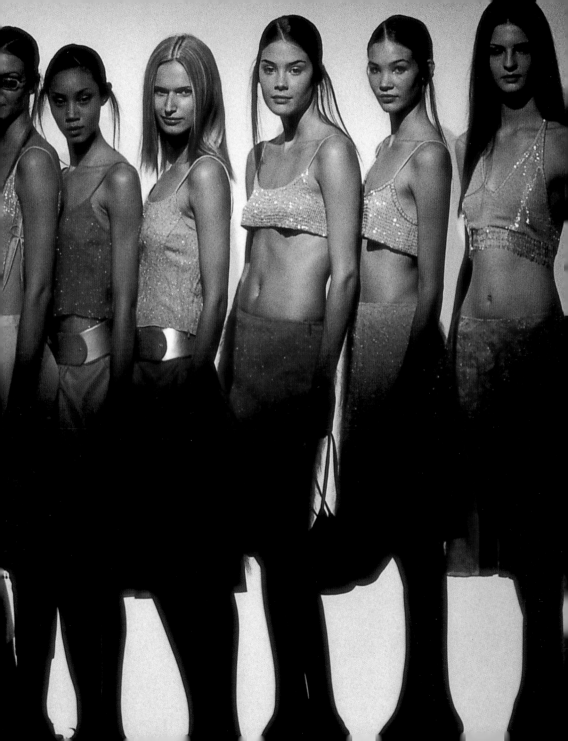

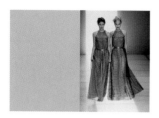

EVENING GRACE

Full-length, spotted, transparent dresses worn belted over strapless bodies, Emporio, Summer 1997.

SHOPPING EXPERIENCE

Restrained Emporio Armani window display, New York 1995.

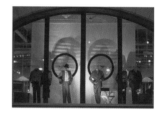

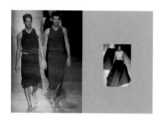

SEPARATES

(Left) soft-striped sarongs worn with singlet vests, Emporio Armani menswear, 1998, and (right) full black skirt worn with cream beaded top for evening, Spring/Summer 1996.

COLOUR

Cerise hipster skirt and matching ruched top, Emporio Armani, Spring/Summer 2000.

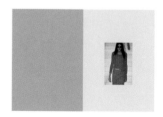

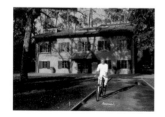

HOME

Giorgio Armani, in casual mode, relaxes at his Milan retreat, 1982.

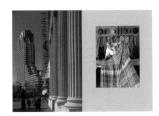

AMERICA/ARMANI

The impressive classical façade of Emporio Armani, (left) San Francisco 1994, and (right) Armani at work, 1982.

ARMANI AT WORK

(Left) a young Giorgio Armani checks the fit of a man's suit on one of his models, 1979. (Top right) Armani puts the finishing touches to a model's make-up. (Bottom right) Armani takes a bow with his models, 1986.

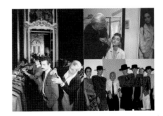

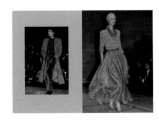

SUIT/ELEGANCE

Collarless grey stripe all-in-one, (left) worn with a soft, broad-shouldered coat, 1984/5, and (right) fluid silk floral print skirt in autumnal hues, multicoloured top, and a bold, peasant-inspired, multi-strand necklace, 1988.

INTRICATE

Indian-inspired evening wear, (left) with a stiffened over skirt decorated with stylized embroidery, 1990, and (right) a sequinned jacket over full-length organza culottes, 1990.

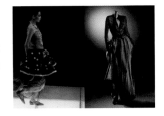

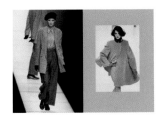

HUES

(Left) signature languid Armani daywear: fine wool, check jacket and contrasting wide-legged, turned-up trousers. (Right) an easy, collarless A-line coat in camel-coloured wool, 1991/2.

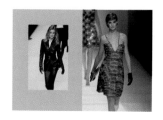

SEXY/SUBTLE

(Left) Surprisingly sexy, yet simple, belted, black leather hotpants suit, Emporio, 1991/2 and (right) characteristically delicate short, beaded halter-neck in subtle aquatic hues, 1992.

WOMENSWEAR/MENSWEAR

(Left) Pared down beige-and-black striped knitted jacket and top, worn with beige trousers, 1992/3 and (right) man's rugged and soft leather jacket, loose striped trousers, waistcoat and sheepskin skullcap, 1993/4.

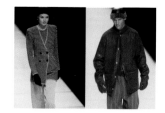

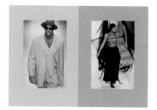

LIGHT AND FLOWING

Signature man's loose and unlined cream linen three-piece suit, (left) 1993 and (right) beaded evening top and black lace skirt, worn with black net veil, 1993.

CLASSIC

(Left) Knee-length red and beige, dog-tooth check jacket worn with contrast pattern waistcoat, Emporio, 1993/4. (Right) single-button, collarless wool crêpe jacket, 1994.

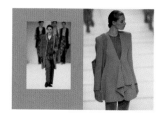

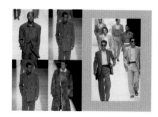

STYLE

(Left) Effortless menswear, 1995/6, and (right) casual summer suits in subtle shades, Emporio and main line collections, 1996.

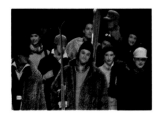

WINTERWEAR

Effortlessly elegant skiwear, Emporio, Autumn/Winter 1995/6.

DAY/NIGHT

Linen shorts suits in natural hues for city wear, (left) Emporio, 1996 and (right) full, black skirt worn with cream beaded top for evening, Spring/Summer 1996.

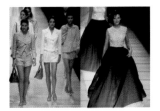

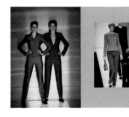

CLEAN-CUT

Fresh and lean, silk trouser suits in rich blues, (left) Emporio, 1996/7 and (right) clean-lined jacket with matching bag, worn with simple, contrasting trousers, Autumn/Winter 1996/7.

ACCESSORIES/TIMELESS

Emporio Armani underwear, and sunglasses and ties for men, (left) Spring/Summer 1997 and (right) an interior and evening wear seen as part of Armani's static still show, Florence, 1997.

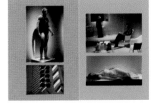

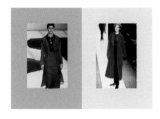

FABRICS

(Left) rich blue, silk chiffon coat and wrap-dress for evening, Spring/Summer 1997 and (right) sumptuous scarlet, wool coat with shawl collar, Emporio, Autumn/Winter 1997/8.

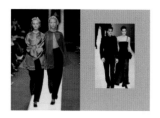

GLAMOUR

(Left) fluid silk 'kimono' tunics in striking colours, Autumn/Winter 1997/8 and (right) sophisticated black evening wear, 1997/8.

SLIMLINE

Restrained opulence for evening, (left) Autumn/Winter 1997/8 and spare, ivory silk, single-button jackets, (right) Spring/Summer 1998.

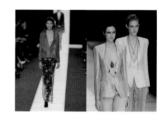

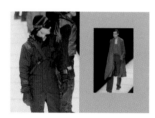

SPORTY/SOPHISTICATED

Skiwear, (left) 1998/9 and distinctive, unstructured, charcoal grey coat (right) with red scarf and shoes, Autumn/Winter 1998/9.

MOVIES/WINONA RYDER AND ARMANI

Richard Gere (top left) in *American Gigolo*, 1980, and (bottom) Sean Connery and Kevin Costner in *The Untouchables*, 1987. Winona Ryder, with Armani, (right) in Armani evening wear.

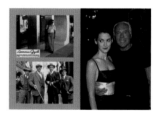

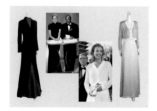

SHARON STONE/EMMA THOMPSON

Sharon Stone, wearing Armani, (left) on stage with Quincy Jones at the 1995 Academy Awards; also present was Emma Thompson, (right) a nominee for best actress in *Sense and Sensibility*.

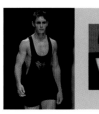

UNDERWEAR/OVERWEAR

Emporio Armani underwear (left) bearing the distinctive stylized Eagle logo, Spring/Summer 1999 and langorous daywear for men, (right) Emporio, Autumn/Winter 1999/2000.

STRIKING

(Left) Appliqué micromini skirt, Emporio, Autumn/Winter 2000/1, with (right) a cerise hipster skirt and matching ruched top, Emporio Armani, Spring/Summer 2000.

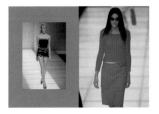

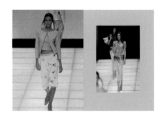

FLUID

Fresh, youthful and languid daywear, (left) Emporio, Spring/Summer 2000 and (right) sheer, sequinned, cut-off trousers and silk top for evening, Spring/Summer 2000.

STUNNING

Emporio Spring/Summer 2000 line-up.

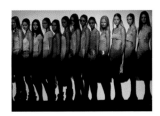

Picture credits

The publishers would like to thank the following sources for their kind permission to reproduce the pictures in this book: